Nutrition Fitness
Copyright © 2020 by Shelia A. Bowens

ISBN: 978-1693083525
Independently Published

On the other side of these next 30 days is a better you. You have the power to live a healthier life. One that is abundantly full. Embrace each challenge because you have the strength to win!!! Establishing a new normal one day, one meal, one exercise at a time.

YOU CAN DO THIS!!!

YOU have the power to live a different life.

Name ____

Age ____________ Gender ____________________

Starting Date ____________ Target Date ____________

Current Weight ____________ Weight Goal ____________

Date	Weight	Time	Notes

Difference:	Goal:

Date __________

<table>
<tr><td colspan="4">DAILY MEAL LOG</td></tr>
<tr><td rowspan="4">BREAKFAST</td><td></td><td colspan="2">SNACK</td></tr>
<tr><td></td><td colspan="2"></td></tr>
<tr><td></td><td colspan="2"></td></tr>
<tr><td></td><td colspan="2"></td></tr>
<tr><td rowspan="4">LUNCH</td><td></td><td colspan="2">SNACK</td></tr>
<tr><td></td><td colspan="2"></td></tr>
<tr><td></td><td colspan="2"></td></tr>
<tr><td></td><td colspan="2"></td></tr>
<tr><td rowspan="4">DINNER</td><td></td><td colspan="2">SNACK</td></tr>
<tr><td></td><td colspan="2"></td></tr>
<tr><td></td><td colspan="2"></td></tr>
<tr><td></td><td colspan="2"></td></tr>
</table>

NOTES

____

____

____

____

OWN YOUR TRUTH BUT PRESS FORWARD.

DAILY MEAL LOG

BREAKFAST		SNACK
LUNCH		SNACK
DINNER		SNACK

NOTES

____

____

____

____

MAKE YOUR FAITH BIGGER THAN YOUR FEAR.

DAILY MEAL LOG

BREAKFAST		**SNACK**
LUNCH		**SNACK**
DINNER		**SNACK**

NOTES

____

____

____

____

SPEAK WHAT YOU WANT TO SEE.

Date ______________

<table>
<tr><td colspan="2" align="center">DAILY MEAL LOG</td></tr>
<tr><td>BREAKFAST</td><td>SNACK</td></tr>
<tr><td>LUNCH</td><td>SNACK</td></tr>
<tr><td>DINNER</td><td>SNACK</td></tr>
</table>

NOTES

____

____

____

____

Date ____________

<table>
<tr><td colspan="2" align="center">DAILY MEAL LOG</td></tr>
<tr><td>BREAKFAST</td><td></td><td>SNACK</td></tr>
<tr><td>LUNCH</td><td></td><td>SNACK</td></tr>
<tr><td>DINNER</td><td></td><td>SNACK</td></tr>
</table>

NOTES

____

____

____

____

YOU MAY STUMBLE. YOU MAY FALL. GET UP!

<table>
<tr><td colspan="2" align="center">DAILY MEAL LOG</td></tr>
<tr><td>BREAKFAST</td><td>SNACK</td></tr>
<tr><td>LUNCH</td><td>SNACK</td></tr>
<tr><td>DINNER</td><td>SNACK</td></tr>
</table>

NOTES

____

____

____

____

WHAT'S YOUR GAME PLAN?

DAILY MEAL LOG

BREAKFAST		**SNACK**
LUNCH		**SNACK**
DINNER		**SNACK**

NOTES

____

____

____

____

SUPPORT IS NOT ALWAYS IN YOUR FACE.

Date __________

DAILY MEAL LOG

BREAKFAST		SNACK
LUNCH		SNACK
DINNER		SNACK

NOTES

____

____

____

____

TAKE YOUR POWER BACK. REMAIN COMMITTED.

Date _____________

DAILY MEAL LOG

BREAKFAST		SNACK

LUNCH		SNACK

DINNER		SNACK

NOTES

____

____

____

____

BE AGGRESSIVELY POSITIVE.

Date _______________

<table>
<tr><td colspan="2">DAILY MEAL LOG</td></tr>
<tr><td>BREAKFAST</td><td>SNACK</td></tr>
<tr><td>LUNCH</td><td>SNACK</td></tr>
<tr><td>DINNER</td><td>SNACK</td></tr>
</table>

NOTES

____

____

____

____

EAT TO LIVE!

Date ____________

<table>
<tr><td colspan="2">DAILY MEAL LOG</td></tr>
<tr><td>BREAKFAST</td><td>SNACK</td></tr>
<tr><td>LUNCH</td><td>SNACK</td></tr>
<tr><td>DINNER</td><td>SNACK</td></tr>
</table>

NOTES

____

____

____

____

LIVE BOLDLY OUT LOUD.

Date _________

<table>
<tr><td colspan="4">DAILY MEAL LOG</td></tr>
<tr><td rowspan="4">BREAKFAST</td><td></td><td colspan="2">SNACK</td></tr>
<tr><td></td><td colspan="2"></td></tr>
<tr><td></td><td colspan="2"></td></tr>
<tr><td></td><td colspan="2"></td></tr>
<tr><td rowspan="4">LUNCH</td><td></td><td colspan="2">SNACK</td></tr>
<tr><td></td><td colspan="2"></td></tr>
<tr><td></td><td colspan="2"></td></tr>
<tr><td></td><td colspan="2"></td></tr>
<tr><td rowspan="4">DINNER</td><td></td><td colspan="2">SNACK</td></tr>
<tr><td></td><td colspan="2"></td></tr>
<tr><td></td><td colspan="2"></td></tr>
<tr><td></td><td colspan="2"></td></tr>
</table>

NOTES

____

____

____

____

ESTABLISH A NEW NORMAL.

Date __________

NOTES

____

____

____

____

THIS STOPS WITH ME!

Date ____________

<table>
<tr><td colspan="2" align="center">DAILY MEAL LOG</td></tr>
<tr><td>BREAKFAST</td><td>SNACK</td></tr>
<tr><td>LUNCH</td><td>SNACK</td></tr>
<tr><td>DINNER</td><td>SNACK</td></tr>
</table>

NOTES

____

____

____

____

Date __________

<table>
<tr><th colspan="2">DAILY MEAL LOG</th></tr>
<tr><td>BREAKFAST</td><td>SNACK</td></tr>
<tr><td>LUNCH</td><td>SNACK</td></tr>
<tr><td>DINNER</td><td>SNACK</td></tr>
</table>

NOTES

____

____

____

____

DAILY MEAL LOG

BREAKFAST		SNACK
LUNCH		**SNACK**
DINNER		**SNACK**

NOTES

____

____

____

____

NEW OPPORTUNITIES ARE FOUND IN EACH DAY.

DAILY MEAL LOG

BREAKFAST		SNACK
LUNCH		SNACK
DINNER		SNACK

NOTES

____
____
____
____

DAILY MEAL LOG	
BREAKFAST	**SNACK**
LUNCH	**SNACK**
DINNER	**SNACK**

NOTES

____

____

____

____

DON'T FORGET TO COUNT THE SMALL VICTORIES.

Date __________

<table>
<tr><td colspan="2">DAILY MEAL LOG</td></tr>
<tr><td>BREAKFAST</td><td></td><td>SNACK</td></tr>
<tr><td>LUNCH</td><td></td><td>SNACK</td></tr>
<tr><td>DINNER</td><td></td><td>SNACK</td></tr>
</table>

NOTES

____

____

____

____

YOU ARE MORE THAN A CONQUEROR!!

DAILY MEAL LOG

BREAKFAST		SNACK
LUNCH		SNACK
DINNER		SNACK

NOTES

____

____

____

____

IT'S IN YOU – PUSH!!!

DAILY MEAL LOG

BREAKFAST		SNACK

LUNCH		SNACK

DINNER		SNACK

NOTES

DAILY MEAL LOG

BREAKFAST		SNACK

LUNCH		SNACK

DINNER		SNACK

NOTES

____

____

____

____

YOUR INNER STRENGTH IS STRONGER THAN YOU THINK.

Date __________

<table>
<tr><td colspan="2" align="center">DAILY MEAL LOG</td></tr>
</table>

BREAKFAST		SNACK
LUNCH		SNACK
DINNER		SNACK

NOTES

____

____

____

____

DAILY MEAL LOG

BREAKFAST		SNACK
LUNCH		SNACK
DINNER		SNACK

NOTES

____

____

____

____

YOU ARE PECULIAR AND THAT'S A GREAT THING.

DAILY MEAL LOG

BREAKFAST		SNACK

LUNCH		SNACK

DINNER		SNACK

NOTES

____

____

____

Date _________

<table>
<tr><td colspan="2" align="center">DAILY MEAL LOG</td></tr>
<tr><td>BREAKFAST</td><td>SNACK</td></tr>
<tr><td>LUNCH</td><td>SNACK</td></tr>
<tr><td>DINNER</td><td>SNACK</td></tr>
</table>

NOTES

____

____

____

____

DON'T BE A SLAVE TO UNPRODUCTIVE THOUGHTS.

Date __________

DAILY MEAL LOG

BREAKFAST		SNACK

LUNCH		SNACK

DINNER		SNACK

NOTES

____

____

____

____

EMPOWERED TO PURSUE IT ALL.

Date ____________

<table>
<tr><td colspan="2" align="center"># DAILY MEAL LOG</td></tr>
</table>

BREAKFAST		SNACK

LUNCH		SNACK

DINNER		SNACK

NOTES

____

____

____

____

QUITTING IS NOT AN OPTION.

Date __________

DAILY MEAL LOG

BREAKFAST		SNACK
LUNCH		SNACK
DINNER		SNACK

NOTES

____

____

____

____